WHAT YOUR NEIGHBORS SAY

DREAM BOOK

Compliments of World's Dispensary Medical Ass'n Buffalo, NY.

Original Edition late 19th century
Dr. Pierce

New Edition 2016
Edited by Tarl Warwick

WHAT YOUR NEIGHBORS SAY – DREAM BOOK

DISCLAIMER AND COPYRIGHT

This work is in the public domain, having been written in the late 19th century. This edition, with its format and cover art, is all rights reserved.

In no way does the editor encourage any of the treatments or advice in this booklet to be used. This text may in no way be construed as able to diagnose, treat, cure, prevent, or ameliorate any disease, condition, symptom, or injury.

WHAT YOUR NEIGHBORS SAY – DREAM BOOK

FOREWORD

This present text is an early edition of one of several infamous quack medicine manuscripts released over time by the late Dr. Pierce, whose medical forays were legendary through the late 19th century and well into the interwar period. In this early period of modern medicine, the fanciful and experimental often coexisted with some degree of peace in the same tracts and in the same medical wards as procedures and philosophies of a more secular, standardized nature. Thus, here, we see an expansive variant of electroshock therapy (notable as having been conducted through most of the building Pierce had built for his "Invalid's Hotel") and the addition of Datura and other potent deliriants to common herbal remedies used even today.

I have omitted, from this edition, the pictures of various folks illustrated in the original text as advocates of Pierce' medicines- these interesting illustrations nonetheless do little other than to show a (possibly fake) face for each patient testimony.

Interestingly, here, a lengthy section on dream interpretation is included with then-modern medical testimonials and folk remedies. That this section is almost a complete plagiarism of the same content from the infamous *Napoleon's Oraculum* circa the 1880s by Tousey is continuing evidence of its lasting power in the burgeoning premodern era of industrialized occultism.

WHAT YOUR NEIGHBORS SAY

High frequency currents are used at the Invalid's Hotel in Buffalo, NY. They promote circulation and increase vitality. They are rich ozone generators, and, when applied yo unhealthy granulations and various skin diseases, act as an oxidizer, antiseptic, and disinfectant. Applied to the skin before incision, they will render the site aseptic.

For general effect the patient is placed upon an auto-conduction couch or in the center of an auto-conduction cage. In the treatment of sub-acute, chronic rheumatism, sciatica, neurasthenia, etc, a condenser couch is most useful.

Write the specialists at Dr. Pierces' Invalids' Hotel in Buffalo, NY., for free, confidential medical advice, no matter what your ailment may be. No charge is made for this service.

WHAT YOUR NEIGHBORS SAY – DREAM BOOK

DREAMS

In most countries and in all ages dreams have been believed in by some people as indications of the future. This form of superstition arises out of the past and present acts of the dreamer. In most ancient days, in Egypt and Babylon, the monarchs' dreams were interpreted by high state officials. The Greeks and the Romans very often consulted the oracles. An inquirer would sleep in the temple at night after performing certain rites, when his questions were supposed to be answered in his dreams.

INTERPRETATION OF DREAMS

ABSENCE: To dream of absent friends means that you will soon hear from them. If they stand near your bed, the news will be bad.

ABYSS: To dream you are looking over an abyss is a warning of danger. To dream that you fall into an abyss denotes illness.

ACCIDENT: To dream that an accident occurs to you means great success. If you see an accident to others beware of false friends.

ANGEL: To dream that you see an angel foretells the death of a beloved friend.

ANIMALS: To dream of domestic animals means a happy return of absent friends and reconciliation of

WHAT YOUR NEIGHBORS SAY – DREAM BOOK

quarrels. Wild animals mean secret enemies.

ANGER: To dream that you have been provoked to anger shows that you have many enemies.

BEAR: To dream that you have seen a bear means you have a rich, cruel, and audacious enemy. If it is running, happiness is in store for you.

BEES: Bees signify wealth and success in business. Seeing bees leave their honey is a sign of honor and fortune.

BEGGAR: If you see yourself a beggar you may hope for wealth. To see many means sickness.

BLOOD: If you see blood, it's a good sign. You will fall heir to riches. To lose blood signifies sorrow and disappointment.

BLOSSOMS: If you see flowers or trees in bloom, it is a sign of success and happiness.

BONNET: For a maiden to dream she gets a new bonnet promises a new lover.

BROTHER: To dream of a brother means an early marriage in your family. If in love, it's a favorable omen.

COW: To dream of a cow means prosperity and abundance.

WHAT YOUR NEIGHBORS SAY – DREAM BOOK

CHILDREN: To see two or three children means that you will have good success in business. To one who has no children to see many children running about the house means it will be difficult for the dreamer to have any.

CLIMBING: To climb a tree means success in life. To climb a steep hill foretells difficulties in life, also sickness.

COFFIN: To see a coffin is unlucky. It means the death of some dear and valued friend.

CRAWLING: This is an ill omen. TO a lover it means a happy marriage.

DANCING: To see dancing is a good omen.

DANGER: To dream of danger is fortunate for you. In business it means success and profit.

DEATH: To dream of death means a wedding. To dream of talking with those who are dead it is a good sign, and you will hear from the living.

DEVIL: It is a sign of sickness and trouble in your family.

DOG: To dream of a dog means your friends are faithful. If he runs behind you, somebody is slandering you. If he fights with another dog, fear persecutions. If he is with a cat, you will quarrel.

WHAT YOUR NEIGHBORS SAY – DREAM BOOK

DROWNING: To dream of this brings happiness; for a woman, a happy marriage.

ELEPHANT: Means riches. To get on his back, good fortune.

FACE: To see a smiling face is a sign of friendship and happiness. A pale face, a sign of trouble and poverty. A black face is a sign of long life.

FALL: To dream you fall from a high place denotes loss of position and goods.

FIRE: To dream you are burnt by fire means you will have a fever. A sparkling fire denotes money in plenty.

FLOWERS: To see them of bright colors means a pleasant life. To see them out of season means bad success. To gather flowers, a lasting friendship. To cast them away, despair and quarrels.

FUNERALS: Good fortune. To attend a funeral, that you will be at a wedding or some gay party.

FLYING: Flying denotes that you will leave your native land and after hardship, return to it rich and happy.

GARDEN: To walk in one means joy, your fortune will be increased.

GRAVE: Means bad success.

WHAT YOUR NEIGHBORS SAY – DREAM BOOK

HILLS: To dream of climbing and traveling over hills signifies good.

HORSES: To dream of horses is a good sign. A white one, unexpected good fortune. To fall from a horse means misfortune and disappointment.

HOUSE: To dream one is building a house means comfort.

HUNGER: Unsatisfied hunger means disappointment in your plans.

HUNTING: If the game is killed, means much trouble through friends, but you discover them and overcome them.

INJURY: To receive an injury means you have many friends. If you dream of causing injury, you will receive and give blessings.

INSULTS: To dream you are abused and insulted means that you will dispute with some person in business.

LETTERS: To write or receive them means good news.

MARRIAGE: To dream of being married signifies death and misfortune. To dream you are present at a wedding of another means joyous news and good luck.

MICE: To dream of mice means prosperity and

WHAT YOUR NEIGHBORS SAY – DREAM BOOK

success in love and a happy marriage.

MISERY: To dream you are in misery and are weeping on account of some calamity or loss means that you will hear good news and that an important change in your affairs will take place.

MONEY: To dream of losing money means loss in business. To find money, if gold, is a good omen. Also to dream of receiving money is good. To dream you lost money is a proof you will be deceived in love. To dream you throw money away means want. To dream of money in bags means misfortune or some kind. Shylock, in the Merchant of Venice, says; "There is some ill abrewing towards my rest, for I did dream of money-bags tonight."

MOTHER: If she be dead, and you dream that you see her living, it is fortunate.

MOUNTAIN: To dream that you see steep, rocky mountains means difficulties in accomplishing your designs.

MURDER: To dream you commit murder warns that you are surrounded by false friends, it signifies danger.

MUSIC: Music means good news.

NOISE: To dream you hear a great noise is a sign of joy. To make a noise, your vanity will be punished.

PURSE: To lose a purse is good. To dream you find

WHAT YOUR NEIGHBORS SAY – DREAM BOOK

a purse or pocketbook full of money is a sign of good luck.

QUARRELS: If one dreams of quarrels and fighting, one will hear of some unlooked-for news or embrace some joy.

RATS: Secret enemies, treason; a sign of having many enemies.

RIDE: To dream you ride with a company of men is very lucky and profitable; with women, it means misfortune and defeat.

RIVER: To dream you see a river, water, clear and calm, means good to all persons. To dream of swimming means future peril and danger.

ROSES: Nothing can be better than to dream of beautiful flowers, if they are in season.

SNAKES or SERPENTS: To see one turning and winding means danger and imprisonment, also sickness and hatred.

SHIPWRECK: To dream you are shipwrecked is dangerous to all.

SHOOTING: To dream you are out shooting is very favorable if you kill much game.

SNOW: Snow is good. To the young it means they will marry and prosper.

WHAT YOUR NEIGHBORS SAY – DREAM BOOK

STORMS: Means a reconciliation.

SICKNESS: Loneliness and imprisonment, tears.

TEARS: If you dream of shedding tears, it means that you will speedily be much happier.

A HEALTHY WOMAN IS ALWAYS BEAUTIFUL

Pittsburgh (North Side) PA: "When I reached middle life I became in a nervous, hysterical condition with despondent spells and frequent heat flashes, also pains in my right side. I took medicines, but not until I took Dr. Pierces' Favorite prescription did I get any relief whatever, but the prescription brought me safely through this critical period just as strong and well as ever.

Doctor Pierces' Favorite prescription is the best medicine in the world for a woman to take throughout this critical period of life" -Mrs. Elmira Bradford, 1202 Palo Alto Street.

Get Doctor Pierces' Favorite prescription at once from your druggist, in either liquid or tablets.

WHAT YOUR NEIGHBORS SAY – DREAM BOOK

THIS ARTICLE WILL INTEREST EVERY MOTHER

Syracuse, NY: "During my young motherhood I had break downs in health. I was nervous and weak and would have such severe backaches that I would not be able to get out of bed for three or four days at a time. I was nauseated and would have dizziness and fainting spells. I was in a miserable condition of health when I began taking Dr. Pierces' Favorite prescription and by the time I had taken two bottles I was well and strong, did not suffer anymore. I kept well and strong up to the last and had practically no suffering." -Mrs. Archie Sutor, 416 Burt. Street.

Send 10 cents to Dr. Pierces' Invalids' Hotel in Buffalo, NY for a trial package. Write for free advice.

BACKACHE OR PAIN OVER KIDNEYS?

Wonderful Relief is Here Told

Toledo, OH: "I was troubled with backache for a year or more. At times, I could hardly bend over to tie my shoes. I lost in weight and worried a lot. I would lose every other days' work. I tried plasters, rubs, and kidney pills, but to no avail. At last my attention was called to Dr. Pierces' Anuric (anti uric acid) tablets, and after using the first bottle I could sleep better and had very little distress. I have used three bottles of this wonderful remedy and I feel like a

WHAT YOUR NEIGHBORS SAY – DREAM BOOK

new man. I recommend anuric to all that I hear complaining of backache, for it certainly did wonders for me." -M.H. Parker, 1213 Jefferson Ave.

This anti-uric acid remedy of Dr. Pierce's for backache and kidneys (called An-Uric) is new, but it can be had at your neighborhood drug store, or send 10 cents for trial package to Dr. Pierce, Invalid's Hotel, Buffalo NY, and write for free medical advice.

A BUSINESS MAN'S ADVICE TO YOU

Health is your Most Valuable Asset

New York, NY: "My business obliges me to go out in all sorts of weather and my health became broken down entirely. Home remedies and doctors did not help me- I tried everything. My joints were sore, stiff, and painful, I had difficulty in going up and down stairs, was constipated, and had stomach trouble. Although I was opposed to put-up medicine, I was willing to take anything. I read of Dr. Pierces' Anuric Tablets and purchased some. Within a few days I felt like a new man, felt like a 'two year old', and still feel so. The Anuric Tablets certainly dig down deep to the very root of one's ailment, and they act very gently and effectively." -C. Robinson, 59 W. 62nd Street.

Don't wait for serious kidney ailment to set in. Help your weakened kidneys with Dr. Pierces' Anuric. Write Dr. Pierce' Invalids Hotel, Buffalo NY for free medical advice.

THE BECKONING LIGHT

By Lillian Lee

It was a dark stormy night, the wind had shifted to eastward, the stars had disappeared under clouds, and within a little fisherman's cottage, on the Newfoundland coast, the good wife feared for her husband's safety, who, she knew, was out on the rough waves with others after mackerel. Outside the storm raged, but within it was warm and cozy, the blazing logs sent ruddy sparks up the wide chimney and beside the fire sat an old woman. At her feet, the house cat slept, and opposite sat a fine buxom young woman, with a beautiful three year old boy in his nightie, all ready for bed. He knelt at his mothers' knee and prayed for daddy's safety, who was out on the wide raging sea, then his mother put a lighted candle in his hand and guided him to the window where he placed it to light the way for daddy, and Donald, seeing the looked-for light, guided his boat to safety and to home.

Women who suffer from ills peculiar to their sex should follow the "beckoning light" to health and happiness by taking Dr. Pierces' Favorite prescription, the famous herbal remedy. It is made from the formula of a skilled physician, of the same herbs and roots long used by the Indians. These women usually are free from feminine disorders and generally pass through the ordeal of motherhood in safety and ease. Dr. Pierce's high standing as a citizen and long experience as a specialist, guarnatees the absolute purity of the Favorite prescription. This is what women everywhere say about it:

Auburn, ME: "Last summer I became ill from feminine trouble, could not work and was very weak all the time. Several doctors failed to cure me- they said the only cure would be by an operation. I began taking Dr. Pierces' Favorite prescription and after taking one bottle I was very greatly improved. Have taken eight bottles, and now weigh 135 pounds, more than I ever weighed before. The 'Prescription' has done wonders for me." -Mrs. Doris Wentworth, 17 Pearl st.

Cleveland, OH: "I take great pleasure in recommending Dr. Pierces' Favorite prescription for any expectant mother, as I have used it myself with great results. My baby is now three months old and I could not wish for a stronger child. My daughter also used it while developing into womanhood." -Mrs. T.H Rogers, 14108 Strathmore Ave.

Rochester, NY: "Through overwork I became all run down in health, was weak and nervous, and suffered a great deal with backaches. I had a tired and worn-out feeling, seemed that I could not get rested, and I was also very nervous. I got Dr. Pierces' Favorite prescription and it did me a world of good. It built me up and gave me strength and my health was very good." -Mrs. E. Beisheim, 667 S. Goodman St.

Favorite prescription is sold by all druggists in liquid or tablet form, or send ten cents for free trial.

USEFUL RECIPES FOR THE HOUSEHOLD

Cleaning Recipes

How to clean brass and copper pans: A piece of cut lemon and coarse salt will clean brass and copper pans like magic. After the pan has been well rubbed, rinse out with clean, warm water, then dry and polish with a dry, soft duster.

To remove grease marks: Grease marks on pages of books may be removed by sponging them with benzine, placing the pages between sheets of blotting paper, and pressing with a warm iron.

Dish cloths: Do not get the attention they should, and in many houses are dirty and quite unfit for use. After washing up, always soap the dish cloth well, and then rinse in hot water with soda in it. Rinse again in hot water, and hang it in the air to dry.

If in Cleaning a kitchen stove the black-lead used is mixed with a little methylated spirit instead of water, the labor of polishing is a good deal reduced and the result is particularly brilliant. Care should be exercised so that the fumes will not ignite.

To remove the smell of onions from knives, place them in the earth for a few minutes. Earth will also sweeten pickle jars, etc, that washing seems powerless to render fit for use, but in that case, the jars should be filled with earth and allowed to remain for twenty four hours or so.

Flower vases stained with flower water can be perfectly cleaned with tea leaves moistened with vinegar.

Your table knives need cause you no anxiety, when stored for some months, if you follow this method; clean the knives thoroughly, and then wipe over with vaseline. Wrap in brown paper, one knife in each fold.

To prevent white fabrics such as tulle or silk evening gowns, choice lace or crepe shawls, becoming yellow when packed away, sprinkle bits of white wax freely among the folds.

To clean carpets: A solution of ammonia and water, lukewarm, will, if well rubbed into carpets, take out all stains. Take one part ammonia to three parts water.

To keep chamois leather soft: The secret of keeping a chamois leather cloth soft is to wash it in warm soap suds, and rinse it in fresh suds (not in clear water), pulling it out periodically while it is hanging up to dry.

Save old kid gloves for ironing day. Sew a pad made from the left glove to the palm of the right one, and you will find your hand is saved from becoming blistered, while the fingers and the back of the hand will be protected from the scorching heat which is so damaging to the skin.

To renovate carpets: Sponge them with a solution of

one part ox-gall to two parts of water; do not make the carpet very wet. Dry thoroughly with clean dusters.

To wash woolen clothes: These should be washed in very hot suds and not rinsed. Luke-warm water will shrink them.

Stained enamel sauce pans should be rubbed with coarse sand and lemon pulp, and not cleansed with boiling soda water. After squeezing lemons, save the pulp for this purpose.

To renovate black kid gloves: Mix together equal quantities of white of egg, black ink, and milk or cream. Put the gloves on the hands and apply the compound to the rubbed parts with a bit of soft flannel. Kid shoes may be treated in the same way.

To restore fur: Heat some rye flour as hot as you can bear your hand on it. Lay this on the fur, let it stand for a quarter of an hour, then shake or brush it out. The fur will be thoroughly cleaned after this process.

To polish windows: A soft newspaper will polish windows and lamp chimneys better than cloth.

To remove stains from garments: Pure chloroform will remove paint, grease, and other stains from colored garments. Put clean blotting paper under the spot and pour the chloroform- a few drops- on it, in the open air.

To remove perspiration stains: Always remove

perspiration stains on white cloths and undergarments in the following manner: First, dampen the article with a little lemon juice before it is put into soap and water.

Silk should never be ironed on the right side, as it will be shiny wherever the iron has touched it.

Smell of paint: To get rid of the smell of paint, let a pail of water stand in the newly painted room.

New Brooms: Soak new brooms in strong hot salt water, before using; this toughens the bristles and makes the brooms last longer.

The economy of brushes is quite worth studying as they quickly mount up to a heavy item in the years' expenditure. A scrubbing brush that is left to soak in a bucket quickly rots. Sweeping brooms should never touch the floor except when in actual use; they should at once be stood on the point of the handle, head upwards, against the wall, if there is not a broomrack. Dusting brushes should have a string on the handle and be hung up after use. Brushes should all be washed from time to time, as they get dirty, just as dusters do.

A suet hint: If suet be melted down in the oven and put into jars, it will keep for any length of time and is much easier to chop up if treated in this way. Puddings will keep better if made from suet that has been melted in the oven.

Never allow meat to remain in paper, or in the kitchen, or it will quickly become tainted.

WHAT YOUR NEIGHBORS SAY – DREAM BOOK

When linen turns yellow after washing, you may know that it has not been rinsed enough. The presence of soap causes the discoloration.

Patent leather shoes should have the dirt removed from them with a damp sponge. Dry with a duster, and then apply a very little vaseline, and polish with a silk handkerchief.

For mildew: Salt, water, and sunshine will remove the worst mildew stains. Wet often, when the sun is bright, and persevere until the garment is clear and white.

Grass stains on leather may be removed by carefully applying benzine or perfectly pure turpentine. Wash the spots over afterward with the well-beaten white of an egg or a good leather reviver.

Frequent dusting saves sweeping. A room that is dusted often and thoroughly will not require such constant sweeping as one that is dusted carelessly and seldom.

Covering a kitchen table: If, when covering a kitchen table with oilcloth, a layer of brown wrapping paper is put on first, it will prevent the oilcloth from cracking and make it wear three times as long.

Old tablecloths when no longer fit for the table, make excellent dress bags. Join up the sides and make a hem top and bottom to take a tape draw-string. If you want to put a delicate skirt away, slip one of these bags over it, and hang in a wardrobe. No dust will then come to it.

WHAT YOUR NEIGHBORS SAY – DREAM BOOK

To clean mirrors: Wash thoroughly with luke-warm water and soap suds, and when dry polish with chamois leather, on which a little finely powdered chalk has been sprinkled.

The bread pan should be washed out weekly, dried, and thoroughly aired by keeping the lid a little way open. Thus, the bread will never get a nasty, musty taste, and to keep it from becoming too dry place a well-washed potato in the pan. Moisture is given off by the potato, but not enough to cause mildew.

A dirty oven is often the cause of a disagreeable smell in the house. The odor may be hard to trace, but try scrubbing out the oven with plenty of soda-water and a brush and the probability is the smell will disappear.

Putting food in the refrigerator: Never put food away in the refrigerator until it is quite cold. Never let anything cool with the lid on. Never leave a metal spoon in any food, even a silver spoon is affected by salt. Never let anything remain all night in a sauce pan- and especially not in enamel ware; many deaths have been caused by neglect of this rule since foods will often become poisoned by being allowed to stand in such cooking utensils. The only really safe receptacle for food to remain in is one of china, glass, or crockery.

Wooden spoons and pastry boards will repay a good scrubbing with sand in preference to soap.

To clean straw matting: Wash with salt and water

and wipe dry. The salt will prevent the matting from turning yellow.

To take out ink stains: If an ink stain gets on your frock, remove it at once with salts of lemon, if the color will not run.

Restoring color to silk: When the color has been taken away from silk by acids, it may be restored by applying to the spot a little hartshorn or sal volatile.

Mending china: To mend china successfully, melt a small quantity of pulverized alum in an old spoon. Before it hardens, rub the alum over the pieces to be united, press them together, and set aside to dry. They will not come apart, even when washed with hot water.

DO YOU NEED A GOOD BLOOD PURIFIER OR TONIC?

If you do, Read This;

Auburn, NY: "My blood was in very bad condition, which caused me to have breaking out all over my body, especially on my limbs and back. I doctored and took medicine, but instead of getting better I grew worse. I got so bad that I had to give up my work, when I decided to try Dr. Pierces' Golden Medical Discovery and by the time I had taken two bottles I was cured of all my trouble. My blood was in a good healthy condition, and I was able to

WHAT YOUR NEIGHBORS SAY – DREAM BOOK

resume my work. I have never had any return of that condition." -Benjamin Kolp, 18 Aspin street.

All druggists, in tablets or liquids.

HAVE YOU A COUGH?

Read What this Woman Says

Elyria, OH: "I can highly recommend Dr. Pierces' Golden Medical Discovery as a household remedy for deep seated coughs and colds and as a tonic and builder in run-down conditions. Golden Medical Discovery has been of great value to me and to my family for years and it is a pleasure to recommend it." -Mrs. Emma Visburgh, 223 Rush st.

When run down you can quickly pick up and regain vim, vigor, vitality, by obtaining this Medical Discovery of Dr. Pierce from your nearest druggist. Send 10 cents to Dr. Pierce, Buffalo NY, for trial package.

WHEN WEAK AND NERVOUS TRY THIS ADVICE

Trenton, NJ: "In my early married life I was rather frail and extremely nervous, and the Favorite Prescription built me up in health and strength and proved to be a splendid nervine. Afterward, I took this same medicine

WHAT YOUR NEIGHBORS SAY – DREAM BOOK

during expectancy as a tonic and strengthener. It was a wonderful help to me all through that trying period and my strength returned rapidly afterward. I have taken Dr. Pierces' Favorite Prescription at various times when run down, weak and nervous, and it has never failed me, therefore I consider it all that could be desired as a tonic and nervine and an excellent medicine for ailments peculiar to women." -Mrs. C.R. Hamilton, 40 Mechanics Ave.

All druggists sell the Prescription in tablets or liquid. Write Dr. Pierce, president Invalid's Hotel in Buffalo NY, for free medical advice.

ADVICE FOR MOTHERS

Mahoningtown, PA: "For several years I have depended upon Dr. Pierces Favorite Prescription to keep me in a healthy condition and it has done me a world of good. I took it before the births of my two youngest children and it kept me free from morning sickness and I felt well and strong, could do all my work and felt fine. Now, whenever I feel weak or in need of a tonic, I take some of the Favorite Prescription and it builds me right up and makes me feel good." -Mrs. George Ae, 504 N. Cedar Street.

Send ten cents for trial package to Dr. Pierce' Invalids Hotel, Buffalo NY.

WHAT YOUR NEIGHBORS SAY – DREAM BOOK

"It is time you 'put your house in order' when you take cold so easily, or are weak from the after-effects of the grip?"

The blood is stagnant and poison accumulates. You show your susceptibility to grip, colds, indigestion and the many ills which accrue from living indoors without proper air and exercise. Feed the body tissues and the organs of the body with good, fresh blood. Bloodless people, thin anemic people, those with pale cheeks and lips, who have a poor appetite and feel that tired, worn, or feverish condition at this time of year, should try the refreshing tonic powers of an alterative and blood purifier. Dr. Pierces' Golden Medical Discovery purifies the blood, stimulates the stomach, and puts the body in the right condition. You feel full of "pep." You have vim, vigor, and vitality after taking this Medical Discovery. This is what folks everywhere testify:

Tioga, PA: "Some years ago I had a severe attack of Grip and was under treatment with one of the best physicians in this part of the country, and, although greatly benefited by his treatment, yet I was left in a miserable condition, nervous prostration seemed to be the leading trouble. I also had bilious headaches and great distress after eating, my stomach would bloat and the least exertion would completely tire me out. I was advised to try Dr. Pierces' remedies and after taking three bottles of the Golden Medical Discovery and three of the Favorite Prescription, also two vials of the Pleasant Pellets, my

health was restored once more. Ever since then whenever I feel run down or in need of a tonic I always take a bottle or two of these medicines with the most pleasing results."
-Mrs. Eney Vanwey Davis, R. D. 3

Alliance, OH: " I take pleasure in stating that I have used the five bottles of Dr. Pierces Golden Medical Discovery, one bottle of the Favorite Prescription, and a vial of the Pleasant Pellets and I am wonderfully improved. I suffered forty years from catarrh. Two years ago I had the flu and suffered from bad head noises and my hearing was impaired. Last September I was so weak I could scarcely walk four blocks away from home, but after giving the Discovery a fair trial, I am now able to sleep about eight hours, also eat a fair meal without suffering indigestion, and can hear the clock tick. I am twenty percent better than I have been for five years." -Mrs. Isabelle Shatalroe.

Druggists sell the Discovery in both liquid and tablets. Send ten cents to Dr. Pierce, Invalid's Hotel, Buffalo NY for a trial package and see for yourself how good it is. Write Dr. Pierce for free medical advice.

HOW TO TELL UNHEALTHY URINE BY ITS APPEARANCE

Unhealthy urine has a greasy, shiny scum on the surface. Blood in the urine is a bad sign.

Color- deep yellow to red, brownish, smoky, or pale

and cloudy.

Consistency: Noticeably thicker than water, heavy.

Less than two and a half pints in twenty four hours, or more than four pints. Too frequent, involuntary, burning or painful, scanty, dribbling, or passage at night.

Odor: Strong, foul, or offensive.

Red brick-dust like sediment, grains like sand, or stringy, whitish settlings.

HEALTHY URINE

Healthy urine is slightly acid but not enough to burn or scald in passing.

Pale yellow to amber color, clear.

Consistency: Scarcely heavier than water.

Three to four pints in twenty four hours, at will during the day, hardly ever at night.

Aromatic or acid, not offensive.

Solid matter: Dissolved, invisible.

It is well to have an urinalysis made occasionally, as kidney disease may be present even though the urine is clear and perfectly normal in appearance.

WHAT YOUR NEIGHBORS SAY – DREAM BOOK

Urine Tested: The Doctor Pierce Clinic of Urology will make a thorough and complete analysis of the urine for the sum of two dollars. This includes a most careful and scientific chemical and microscopical examination, also a bacteriological stain of the sediment, if indicated, and a complete type-written report of the analysis, with a letter of explanation, will be sent to you by return mail. We will furnish a mailing case for sending sample (approved by the United States Post Office Department) with bottle and preservative, and send same mail for two times.

This is a service of which a great many people are taking advantage today. It helps to keep tabs on your general health, and may prolong life. Many of our patrons have an analysis made regularly, every three months.

Whens ending sample for analysis write us under separate cover, giving a statement and history of your case. Ask any medical questions you wish answered.

Address: Dr. Pierces' Invalids Hotel
665 Main Street, Buffalo NY.

DAINTY DISHES FOR THE INVALID

Barley Water: One and a half tablespoons peal barley, one quart cold water, salt. Wash barley, add cold water and let soak several hours or overnight. Drain and add the fresh cold water, boil gently over direct heat two hours, or in a double boiler steadily four hours, down to one pint, adding water from time to time; season with salt Strain through muslin. Cream or milk may be added or lemon juice and sugar.

Rice Water: Two tablespoons rice, one pint cold water, salt, milk. Wash and pick over the rice; add cold water and cook until rice is tender. Strain and dilute with boiling water or hot milk to desired consistency. Season with salt. Sugar may be added if desired, and cinnamon, if allowed, may be cooked with it, and will assist in inducing a laxative condition.

Oatmeal Water: One tablespoon oatmeal, one tablespoon cold water, a speck of salt, one quart boiling water. Mix oatmeal and cold water, add salt, and stir into boiling water. Boil three hours; replenish the water as it boils away. Strain through cheese cloth. Season, serve cold.

Junket: One cup fresh milk, one quarter Junket tablet, one teaspoon cold water. Heat the milk until lukewarm, add the tablet dissolved in the cold water; allow it to jelly in a warm place; chill in a cool place.

Flaxseed Tea: One tablespoon whole flaxseed, two cups cold water, juice of one lemonl sugar. Wash flaxseed thoroughly, put it with the cold water in a sauce pan, simmer one hour, add lemon juice and sugar to taste and strain. If too thick, add hot water. Valuable in case of inflammation of the mucous membrane.

Egg Broth: Yolk one egg, one tablespoon sugar, a speck of salt, one cup hot milk. Brandy or some other

WHAT YOUR NEIGHBORS SAY – DREAM BOOK

stimulant if required. Beat egg, add sugar and salt. Pour on carefully the hot milk. Flavor as desired, if with brandy or wine use about one tablespoon.

Egg-Nog: One egg, a speck of salt, one tablespoon sugar, one third cup of milk, one and one half tablespoons of wine or less of brandy. Beat the egg, add the sugar and salt, blend thoroughly, add the milk and liquor. Serve immediately.

THE EXPERIENCE OF A PROMINENT MAN

Chester, PA: "I was taken with rheumatism in my right knee. I could not walk for ten days, and had to use a crutch or a stick for more than two months. After trying different remedies and getting no relief I saw an advertisement of Dr. Pierces' Anuric Tablets. I bought two bottles and before I had taken half a bottle I could walk without a stick. I continued to take them until I had taken nearly two bottles (dieting myself as directed) and I was well. My knee has given me no more trouble since." -W.M. Bell, 1115 Upland St.

HOW ARE YOUR KIDNEYS?

Lewiston, PA: "I had the flu and it seemed to have affected my kidneys. I had terrible headaches and pain in my back from which I was not relieved until I took Dr.

WHAT YOUR NEIGHBORS SAY – DREAM BOOK

Pierces' Anuric Tablets. I had taken only part of a ottle until I was relieved. I also find them very beneficial for colds. I have taken Dr. Pierces' Golden Medical Discovery and the Favorite Prescription too with fine results." -Mrs. Dewey Hoffman, R.D. 4

Help your weakened kidneys by obtaining this Anuric (anti-uric acid) of Dr. Pierces' at your nearest drug store or send ten cents for trial package to Dr. Pierce' Invalids Hotel in Buffalo NY.

YOUR GOOD HEALTH AND LONG LIFE DEPEND ON YOUR KIDNEYS

Salamanca, NY: "Last spring my feet and ankles started to swell terribly. I could not wear any shoes and by afternoon could scarcely walk around at all. I thought it must be caused from my kidneys so I got a bottle of Dr. Pierces' Anuric Tablets, and before the bottle was gone my ankles and feet had stopped swelling. I took three bottles of the tablets and now feel fine. I am so thankful for the benefit I derived from this wonderful remedy of Dr. Pierce's that I tell of it whenever I get the chance." -Mrs. Lewis Dickerson, 38 Elm St.

Bennettsburg, NY: "I had kidney trouble, also neuritis in my arms, hands, and feet. They would pain so I could not sleep nights until I took Doctor Pierces' Anuric

Tablets, and was entirely cured." -Mrs. Bert Bailey, Box 61.

You can quickly put yourself in A-1 condition by going to your druggist and obtaining Dr. Pierces' Anuric Tablets or write Dr. Pierce, president Invalid's Hotel in Buffalo NY for free confidential advice. Send ten cents for trial package.

BEAUTY IS SKIN DEEP

Good Blood is Beneath Both

Harrison, NY: "For years I was bothered with my blood and stomach and also constipation. The doctor said I was anemic and if I didn't take care of myself he feared consumption. His medicine failed, so my mother decided to try the remedies she had used for ten or twelve years. She started to give me Dr. Pierces' Golden Medical Discovery, a good blood tonic, and Dr. Pierces' Pleasant Pellets for my bowels, and these medicines made me feel fine. I was not able to sleep nights and was irritable before, but after taking the Discovery, I could sleep well and felt good. I thought my case was hopeless, and I was cured so you may be, too. Why suffer?" -Mrs. H. Doen, East White Plains.

Your neighborhood druggist carries a full line of Dr. Pierces' famous remedies. Write Dr. Pierce, president, Invalid's Hotel, in Buffalo NY for free medical advice. Send ten cents if you desire a trial package of any of Dr. Pierces' remedies in tablet form.

WHAT YOUR NEIGHBORS SAY – DREAM BOOK

DR. PIERCES' FAMILY MEDICINES

Mailed directly by Dr. Pierces' Laboratory in Buffalo, NY, on receipt of price, if not kept by your neighborhood druggist.

DR. PIERCES' GOLDEN MEDICAL DISCOVERY is an alterative and vegetable tonic. Contains no alcohol. Tablets, small size; 65 cents. Large size; $1.35. Liquid; $1.35.

DR. PIERCES' FAVORITE PRESCRIPTION is an herbal tonic for chronic weaknesses of women. Contains no alcohol, nor any harmful ingredient. Tablets, small size; 65 cents. Large size; $1.35. Liquid; $1.35.

DR. PIERCES' ANURIC TABLETS A new remedy for kidney, bladder, and uric acid troubles. Price, 65 cents. Large size, $1.35.

DR. PIERCES' IRONTIC (iron-tonic) TABLETS: Makes redder blood. Price, 65 cents.

DR. PIERCES' PLEASANT PELLETS for constipation, billious and sick headaches, indigestion and many derangements of the stomach, liver, and bowels, when due to constipation, are corrected by their use. Price, 30 cents.

DR. PIERCES' COUGH SYRUP: for coughs, colds, hoarseness, bronchial coughs and non-diptheric sore throat. Price, 30 cents.

DR. PIERCES' HEALING SALVE: A nice dressing for open, running, or suppurating sores and ulcers. Price, 65 cents.

DR. PIERCES' ANODYNE PILE OINTMENT: A soothing, cooling, healing antiseptic application for piles. Price, 65 cents.

DR. PIERCES' SOOTHALINE (Mentha): Especially recommended for sunburn, chilblains, tired burning aching feet, chapped skin. Applied after shaving, this Soothaline is very cooling and healing. Price, 65 cents.

WHAT YOUR NEIGHBORS SAY – DREAM BOOK

FIRST AID TO THE INJURED

Apoplexy: Apply wet cloths to the head and open the collar. Give a laxative.

Bites of Snakes, Mad Dogs, etc: Apply a ligature (a cord) on the side nearest the heart; suck the wound. Scratch the edges with a clean penknife, and apply caustic or carbolic acid to the wound.

Stings of Insects: Apply weak ammonia, oil, salt, water iodine.

Burns and Scalds: Cover with cooking soda and lay wet cloths over the injured part. Apply white of egg and olive oil; olive or linseed oil, plain or mixed with chalk and whiting; sweet or olive oil and lime water.

Fainting: Place flat on back; allow fresh air, and sprinkle with water. Place head lower than the rest of the body.

Fire from Kerosine: Don't use water, it will spread the flames. Dirt, sand, or flour is the best extinguisher. Or smother with a woolen rug, tablecloth, or carpet.

Fire in a Building: Crawl on the floor. The clearest air is the lowest in the room. Cover head with woolen wrap, wet if possible. Cut holes for the eyes. Don't get excited.

Fire in One's Clothing: Don't run; especially not down stairs or out of doors. Roll on carpets, or wrap in woolen rug or blanket. Keep the head down so as not to inhale flame.

Fits: Loosen the clothing about the neck, admit plenty of fresh air, and prevent the patient from injuring himself. Place a cork between the jaws to prevent patient from biting his tongue.

Sprains and Strains: There is nothing better than Dr. Pierces' Ammonio-Camphorated Liniment. It penetrates to the strained muscles and tendons so that the pain and inflammation subsides.

Sunstroke: Loosen clothes at neck; administer a laxative; apply cold water to the head.

DR. PIERCES'
Invalids Hotel and Surgical Institute

665 Main Street, BUFFALO, NY

(Incorporated by special act of the New York Legislature)

Organized with a full staff of physicians and surgeons for the treatment of chronic diseases.

PIERCES' PLEASANT PURGATIVE PELLETS

Are composed of may-apple (podophyllin), Jalap, Aloin, and Extracts of Nux Vomica and Stramonium in minute quantities. These Pleasant Pellets operate without disturbance to the system, diet or occupation. Put up in glass vials, and sold by all druggists. Always fresh and reliable. As a laxative, or gently acting cathartic, these little Pleasant Pellets give good satisfaction.

Send ten cents for trial package to Doctor Pierces' Invalids Hotel, 665 Main Street, Buffalo NY.

www.ingramcontent.com/pod-product-compliance
Lightning Source LLC
Chambersburg PA
CBHW070340190526
45169CB00005B/1974